I Don't Know How to Give Up

Lucky to live with Type 1 Diabetes:

My Story

Caridad Cachupin

Copyright Notice

Copyright © 2026, Caridad Cachupin

All rights reserved. No part of this publication may be copied, reproduced, republished, translated, stored, or transmitted in any form or by any means—whether electronic, mechanical, digital, or otherwise - without the prior written permission of the publisher.

This book is the result of dedication, creativity, and countless hours of effort. Any resemblance to real persons, living or dead, is purely coincidental—or perhaps just the universe having a bit of fun.

Published by Kinetic Digital Publishers

www.kineticdigitalpublishers.com

For permissions, inquiries, or other correspondence, please visit our website.

Paperback ISBN: 979-8-90235-068-2

Hardcover ISBN: 979-8-90235-069-9

eBook ISBN: 979-8-90235-067-5

LCCN: 2026903420

DEDICATION

I would like to dedicate this book to the most valuable thing that a mother has, my sons Brian and Kevin, and to my husband, my life partner. I would also dedicate this book to my adoring parents who always protect me from heaven. Likewise, my students are a source of inspiration and positive energy in my life.

TABLE OF CONTENTS

Introduction..3

Chapter 1... 4

   The Surprise 4

Chapter 2 9

   Honeymoon..9

Chapter 3 12

   Your Mental Health..12

Chapter 4... 17

   Nutrition..17

Chapter 5 22

   Your Physical Activity 22

Reflection..28

I Don't Know How to Give Up

The day is today, live it intensely. Tomorrow is uncertain. Enjoy every second as if it were your last. Don't worry about the future. Inevitably, what you have predestined will happen. Nothing is going to stop you from escaping your fate.

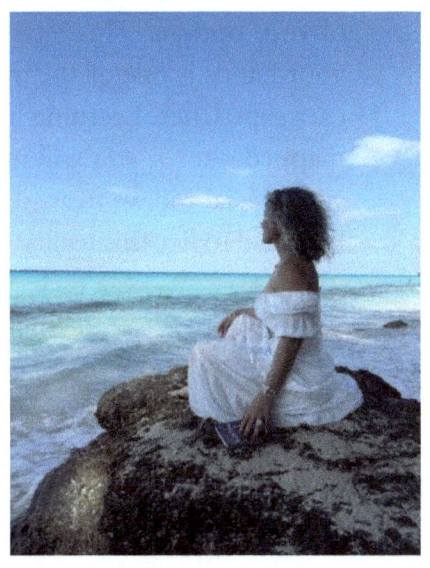

There will be many things that you will incorporate into your life and it is okay that way because each day will be unique and unrepeatable. Being diabetic does not allow you rest, your mind will always be busy counting carbohydrates, attending to your constant highs and lows of sugar among other things. What for others might be a normal routine day, will not be for you so you will have to get used to never getting bored. Sweets are never going to be pampered after a busy day. You will always have these available, but not for when you feel like it, but for when you need them. They could really help you get out of a not-so-pleasant time. Every night of sleep and rest makes you rethink what you could have done better so as not to repeat the mistakes of the previous day. Your alarm will wake you up in the middle of the night that more than annoying us we appreciate the enormous blessing of having a guardian angel watching our backs.

This precious liquid called insulin will save your life many times but at the same time it could be your most dangerous tool. Many times you will feel in an abyss that you will have to fight again and again, you see that it is not your time, that there are many battles to win and show everyone that giving up is not one of your options. This bittersweet feeling of having your life in your hands is one of the most overwhelming feelings you will ever experience. Learning how to challenge this destiny already mapped out for you will make you stronger every day. We are very special and we treasure moments that only those of us who have had to live this reality understand.

Join me to unravel this paradoxical skein that many may not understand but that is a reality for millions of people around the world."

Introduction

You will think, who can feel lucky to suffer from such a disease? That person is crazy. I just want to make you reflect so that you understand that not everyone can tell their story, and those are already points in my favor. Every day is a gift from God, even if most of the time we don't see it that way. I feel like a lucky person because, despite the difficulties I face every day, I am here alive to watch the sun rise every morning, watch my children grow up, and thank God for every second of my life. Many times, we think "because of me," but we don't think it could have been worse.

Each and every one of the things that have happened to me in my life, whether good or bad, I have learned to see the positive side of them. This has helped me to see life from another point of view and has made me feel better. Many things have happened to me that I don't think I deserved, but these, in turn, taught me that I was stronger than I thought. Remember that God will take people or things away from you for your protection, but He will leave many more for your training. The things that go away, let them go, and the things that stay, let them be, even if they are not to your liking. I hope I can help you change those negative thoughts that will help you face life with a different attitude.

Something very positive that I thank for the education I had since I was a child is that I have become a very disciplined person in all aspects of my life. Like everyone else, I like to enjoy the pleasures of life, but I learned that all things have to be measured because no excess is good.

Chapter 1

The Surprise

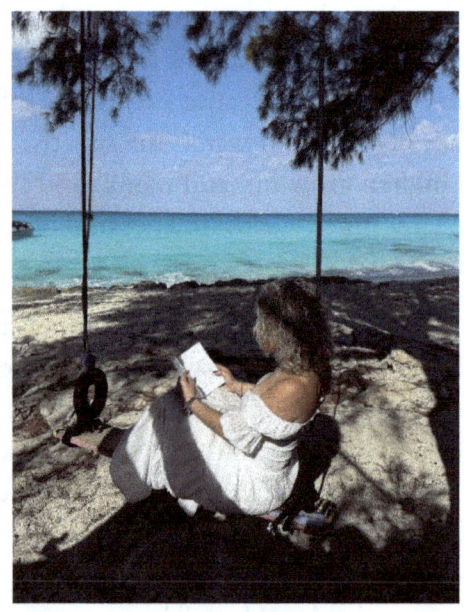

My life went on like that of any ordinary person. As usual, I followed my eating and exercise routine because I have always liked to look and feel good. I took very good care of my sleep hours and always tried to stay away from things that hurt me. Every year, when I had my annual exam, the doctor told me to keep doing what I did because I was 15 despite being over 40. This motivated me to continue the healthy lifestyle that I am used to following. My exercise routine was very intense, but I noticed that despite working hard with my muscles, they didn't grow enough as they should have, considering that I was doing CrossFit, but I didn't give it much importance, despite thinking about it, because I don't like to look muscular.

Everything was going well; there was nothing to complain about. Every summer, I have my annual check-up, and as always, it was good. I even thought about not doing it that year, but in the mornings for two or three days when I woke up, I felt dizzy, which passed as the day went by. I never thought anything was wrong; I just thought I had overdone it in some weight exercise, and my cervical was feeling it. It never crossed my mind that it could be something else. I said, it's going to happen, I'm just going to decrease the weight in some of my exercises. So the days went by, and I even felt better and thought the problem was solved. The next week, the dizziness recurred, and I even felt that something different was happening inside my body: it was the sensation of a herd of horses trotting inside me. I changed my mind and decided to have the annual checkup. To my surprise, the doctor tells me, you have altered sugar, and I thought that's what I did the tests the day after returning from a cruise, which we know is usually eaten much more than normal.

The doctor told me that he sent me pills to lower blood sugar levels, and that was it. That did not convince me because I have never liked to take medicines; usually, all my discomforts were solved with exercises, and I thought I was going to look for a specialist, and that is what I did. If I had listened to the first doctor who prescribed me pills, it would have been a total failure that would only have affected my body even more, so I got a second opinion. I started researching what would be the best endocrinologist in Miami. I ended up finding a team of endocrinologists at the University of Miami Lenar Foundation research center, who were very special to me, and started the research.

When the doctors told me that one of the antibodies to diabetes was indeed altered, I couldn't believe it. How many questions came to my mind? Why has this happened? What did I do wrong if all I do is lead a healthy life? What good has everything I've done for years been me? I absolutely could not have taken pills because type one diabetes does not require it; I was even happy not to have heard the first medical opinion. Still, I believed that somehow I was going to be able to cure my illness.

Here began my search for explanations that I want to share with you. The doctors told me at that time that this type of Type 1 diabetes is mostly hereditary, contrary to what they say, no, that it is caused by a very strong stress that causes the gene for diabetes that we all fear inside, as well as that of cancer and other diseases, to be activated. My questions and concerns continued. Where did it come from if neither of my parents had diabetes, not even I had it during my two pregnancies? This type of diabetes develops in children, mainly not in adults like me. At my age, I could suffer from type 2 diabetes due to poor diet, being overweight, etc., but this is not my case, as always, wanting to know everything, I began to investigate my ancestors more. Of my two paternal grandparents, both had died at an advanced age from other diseases unrelated to diabetes, and my maternal grandparents, my grandmother died at the age of 86 from other reasons unrelated to diabetes, and my grandfather? What happened here with my paternal grandfather, who never even saw a picture of himself? What happened to 'Daddy?' That was what my mother called him.

My grandfather died when my mother was 11 years old. My grandmother raised her alone, and years ago, it was not very common to be portrayed like this. I thought that was the reason why I never saw a photo of him. Also, my mother had very few memories of him because at 11 years old, there is not much we can remember. My mother told me that grandfather had died because he had fallen from his feet and hit his head badly, and that was his cause of death. There were no autopsy results or any suspicion that anything else had happened to grandfather. I begin to draw my own conclusions: grandfather has either hypoglycemia or hyperglycemia, both of which are fatal. As they did not know that they suffered from any disease, this was the conclusion they gave to his sudden death; he hit himself in a bad place on the head. Since no one knew what was happening, there was no medical intervention, and so grandfather's life ended.

Bingo, I think this is where the water comes into the coconut. Genetics does not fail; no matter what you do, if your body is genetically predisposed to a disease, it will simply give you. It is also useless to blame your family member because they also inherited it from someone else. No one is to blame; it's simply what you have to live with, whether you like it or not.

On the other hand, if it is not genetic, what happened? Like all living beings on this planet, situations happen to us for which we are not prepared, and without a doubt, they cause us a lot of stress, or we would say suffering that, believe it or not, hurts each and every one of your organs, although if they told me at that time I did not understand it in any way. My life was so engrossed among so many of these problems that how could I imagine that, in addition to these problems that overwhelmed me so much, my own body was also going to attack me, bringing me any kind of disease. I couldn't even imagine that. My mother, the person who has loved me the most and I have loved in life, was going through a very serious degenerative disease, and it was not under me to make her feel better, much less cure her. This, among other things, affected my whole life in every way, my marriage, my work, and even my children, who indirectly suffered with me, joining everything like a time bomb ready to explode inside me at any moment.

Sometimes we believe that we are super powerful, that nothing will stop us, we believe we are super women, super moms, or super wives, that we are in control of everything and that we will solve everything by ourselves without anyone's help, but believe me, that it is a complete mistake and we do not realize it until we are discarded. Absolutely everything can wait; things don't have to be perfect. I recommend you to seek a balance between the role of mother/wife and woman, cultivate couple and personal relationships, and not sacrifice your own professional and personal goals and above all not sacrifice our health because once we lose it, all the sacrifices made previously were worth nothing if we cannot enjoy it as we should later. It is necessary to understand that asking for help is not a sign of weakness, but of intelligence. You can delegate tasks to your partner or other family members. We can express our needs clearly and communicating our own feelings and limitations is essential for our physical and emotional well-being. It is important to set aside time for yourself, to enjoy personal activities, or simply to rest and recharge. Maintaining hobbies and self-interests outside of the family and professional sphere helps to maintain individual identity and happiness.

Chapter 2

Honeymoon

Unlike type 2 diabetes, in which many people are overweight, their bodies are able to produce insulin, which is not properly distributed. Type 1 diabetes: My pancreas does not produce the insulin that my body needs and that is why it needs to be delivered subcutaneously. My immune system, for some reason, attacks the cells of the pancreas and does not let them produce insulin, and that is why we become insulin-dependent. Type 2 diabetes, according to some articles with which I do not agree, is supposedly reversible following an adequate exercise and diet regime, but I particularly do not think so, because once you decide to stop exercising or eating what you should not in excess, you go back; that does not mean that you are cured, so I particularly do not believe that it has a cure as stated by many articles and programs that sell you a supposed miracle cure which does not exist, so why let ourselves be deceived.

All this chemical imbalance that was happening in my body caused me to lose weight or muscle mass because I really don't have fat in my body, so in this way, my muscles are the ones that are affected. This is called ketoacidosis, which happens when sugar levels are continuously high for a certain time and the body uses your fats to produce energy. This process produces acid in your blood called ketones that can be very dangerous and can even cost you your life and require immediate medical attention. You can imagine how stressful and frustrating it was for me because for the first time, I felt like I didn't have control over my body. On the other hand, I was very lucky to meet doctors who were very patient with me, helping me answer so many questions that I couldn't find the meaning or answers to. A great help to understand what was happening to me was the internet, where you don't always find the right answers, but it is a great source of information, always available to everyone with a single click. That is why I decided to write my story so that it can help someone else clarify their ideas and make them feel that they are not the only ones, that there are millions of people who have the same condition but with the right aptitude, the help of professionals, and the support of your family, you will be able to, like me, feel grateful to live with type 1 diabetes because unlike other diseases this is not the only one. It takes your life in one fell swoop but gives you the opportunity to depend largely on yourself.

For two years, I was using vitamins that helped me decrease the inflammation in my pancreas, and that way, I could produce some of the insulin that my body needed. After two years, my honeymoon with the diabetes, as the doctor calls it, was over. Now I was going through the bad things, and these vitamins that definitely helped me for a while did not want to work anymore. You will never be better every day; as a result of the aging of your body, your pancreas will want to work less, to put it in a simple way, and that you can understand better, and that is why you will have to use greater amounts of insulin as time goes by. In addition, when you start supplying insulin subcutaneously, your body reacts in the following way: if they are giving me what I need, I will not produce it anymore, and that is how the little production you had, so to speak, stops

being provided by your pancreas, and in this way you are at the mercy of your own decisions to supply this valuable medicine, and I say valuable because without it we could not live. Now begins the stage of understanding how we count each and every one of the carbohydrates we eat to try to supply us with the correct dose of insulin. I say the correct one, although it is never the same. Every day, your body has different needs, but you will have to learn to know yourself. Every day is a constant struggle to try to guess the best decision for each day. However, this really doesn't matter to me; I'm going to continue to fight to be and feel better.

It's been tough times, a constant struggle one day at a time. Every day has been different. What works for you today may not work for you tomorrow even if you do the same thing. Unfortunately, you learn with the blows of everyday life living with the disease, but if I can help you with my advice in this process, that will make me feel better. If I tell you that it is easy, I would be lying to you, but I can tell you that 50% is on your side, and the other 50% are many other things that I will explain shortly. It depends a lot on you to want to see and feel better.

Three factors that guarantee the success of a healthy life with type 1 diabetes are:

1- Your Mental Health.

2- Your diet.

3- Your physical activity.

The balance of these three important aspects is decisive for your quality of life to be optimal. Below, I will help you with valuable insights that I have learned over time, living with the disease, which have been useful to improve my quality of life and balance my blood sugar levels.

Chapter 3

Your Mental Health

You can see that my number 1 factor is mental health. This, in my opinion, is the most important because you could eat well and do physical activity, but if your mind and soul are not calm and at peace, nothing will work properly. You may be wondering, but how do I achieve that balance with so many challenges that life puts in my path every day? My answer is to have a positive attitude no matter how stressful your day is, look for the moment when you can pause in the midst of the chaos and get closer to God and ask Him to give you the serenity you need to continue your day, to help you overcome your fears and insecurities, to take away the stress that does not let you feel good. Talk to Him, He always listens to you, even if you don't believe it, even if you don't see it. He's there looking at you through the eyes of maybe a bird or someone else. Whenever you ask Him from the bottom of your heart, He will always listen to you.

Accepting that you have a medical condition that you are going to live with for the rest of your life is very important. Don't blame anyone, don't let them see you with pity, and don't expect someone to come and do for you what only you have the power to do. No one owes you anything or owes anyone anything. Yes, you are going to have limitations, but in your mind. When you change your mind and order her that you can and that nothing and no one is going to stop you, you will begin to see how you are definitely going to achieve your goals. Easy is not the one who said that life is easy, but you have to learn to be strong because this is your only option. All people face numerous difficulties and challenges on a daily basis, you are not the only person who faces extreme situations in which, without expecting it or even worse, without having done anything to deserve it, terrible things happen to them.

Don't give up. Never accept the role of defeat. Learn to overcome your fragility. Be strong and never accept the victim's dialogue because you are not. Always think that it could have been worse and that you are here telling your story. I know there will be difficult days, but don't forget that you can't give up. If today your day was not the best, it doesn't matter, think that tomorrow will be different, but keep trying. Love life and love yourself above all things. We are not perfect, and we certainly make many mistakes, but we can create goals and change our attitude and aptitude because these are going to define our lives. Do not give up in the face of difficulties because this is just one of the many adversities that life has prepared for you. Do not give up, fight intensely, and put all your passion and dedication into what you want to achieve in life. Remember that you only have one life to try, and on my part, they will not say that at least I did not try with all the claws and energies I could. If you want to, take it as proof of life so that you never forget how vulnerable we are, that life can change you in a second, but you have to be prepared to face it with dignity, drive, and determination.

Dignity because you can never allow someone to underestimate you because something is not right with your health. Show them what you're made of and don't accept a "you can't" as an answer. Push because you are the guide of your life and your destiny and the more you put in the effort and don't let yourself give up, the further you will go in your life. Determination, because when you set a goal and have a firm goal and a purpose to live for, you are going to be absolutely unstoppable; nothing is going to stop you, even if it is the last thing you do in life.

Honor your life. You have made it worth living. Not to be remembered for the failures you have had, but for your infinite perseverance, to try incessantly, to never give up until you achieve your purpose. In this specific case, it is to achieve quality of life. That your bad actions or determinations related to your health do not lead you to have more serious complications later in your health, as you know that diabetes has. Your family plays a huge role in your emotional balance. I was lucky enough to grow up in a large family where we didn't have much financially but I always had the love of my parents and my siblings.

Unfortunately, nothing is eternal; your parents grow old and leave, and the other people you thought were always going to be there are not there, but life and God reward you with people you never imagined would be by your side, supporting you in every triumph and every failure. I am blessed to have two princes who are the engines of my life and a marriage that, although not perfect like any other, has been a blessing in my life; we have grown together and overcome many difficulties, as well as shared many unforgettable moments.

I have many friends who I consider family that are not there, and so I have achieved emotional balance with those who I consider to be my true family. Certainly, you are going to lose people who are important to you, as well as many others will enter your life, but just welcome those who arrive, thank you to those who are there and those who leave, just bless them, but do not let other people's decisions affect your life, people like many other things come and go. Not always will what you think is right be for everyone. Always do what you believe is right, and don't worry about what they will say; you will not always look good with everyone.

At work, always do what you are passionate about doing. Remember that you have to go to work every day. Imagine always doing something that makes you uncomfortable. If you're not happy, change it. Once you feel happy doing what you like to do every day, your body and your sugar levels will thank you. You will feel the change immediately. I know it could be difficult, as it was for me to finally do what I like in the right place, but don't stop trying every day to be able to place yourself in that desired place.

In this moment of vulnerability, it's important to acknowledge the emotional toll that living with Type 1 diabetes can take. It's okay to feel this way, to question, and to wonder why, because it's part of the journey. Through all of it, remember: You are not alone, and you have the strength to continue.

Caridad Cachupin

Dear pancreas, what have you done?
Have you forgotten about me?
With how well I have treated you,
For you to do this to me.
Suddenly you decided
to stop doing your job,
and without finding a shortcut,
I set out to replace you
from the very bottom.
Oh my child, what wouldn't I do
to make you work again,
to cuddle you like
a little baby
and put all my faith
that soon you will be back.
I should be angry
because you really failed me,
but you also taught me
to live day by day
and to understand that life
sometimes brings surprises,
but you have to face them
with the best strength.
And here I am without you,
with my body full of holes,
longing for that past
which I hope returns soon.

Chapter 4

Nutrition

I've always heard it said that we are what we eat and there's a lot of reason in this. This disease requires a lot of dietary discipline. The power of your mind plays a fundamental role in you. The first thing you have to change, either to lose weight or to take care of your diabetes, is your mind. Dominate it, don't let it do it with you. You have the power to choose what is best for you. Nowadays, there are many temptations to which you have to learn to say no. Supermarkets are loaded with highly processed foods that are poisonous not only for you living with the disease, but for each and every human being. Create habits that help you control your sugar levels.

Fortunately, we have a lot of food. Take control of your health and well-being. Fruits and vegetables, whole grains such as wheat, brown rice, quinoa, and oatmeal. Also, proteins such as lean meats, chicken, turkey, fish, eggs, nuts, beans, and lentils. In addition, low-fat or low-fat products such as milk, yogurt, and cheese, consumed properly and in the correct portions, are very healthy for your diet. Alcoholic beverages are not highly recommended if you live with diabetes. I particularly recommend a good wine to accompany meals or celebrations. This neither raises nor lowers your sugar levels and, unlike other drinks such as tequila, perhaps when you are eating and you accompany it with a few drinks it will even help you lower your levels a little, but then you will have the rebound effect the next day and on most days you will wake up on an empty stomach with this high product of the intake the day before of Tequila.

On the contrary, wine is not going to make you feel bad the next day. So I personally recommend it, obviously in moderation.

Let's Start with Breakfast

A great option is low-sugar, low-fat yogurt, because not all of them are the right ones; you have to look at the labels. I, in particular, consume a Greek yogurt with 2 grams of sugar per 6-ounce serving with nuts such as granola seeds, pumpkin, almonds, quinoa, and amaranth, among others. You don't have to consume them all at once; you can intersperse different ones every day, so you don't bore yourself. You could also have whole wheat or seed bread for breakfast with salmon and cured cheese, as well as dark chocolate.

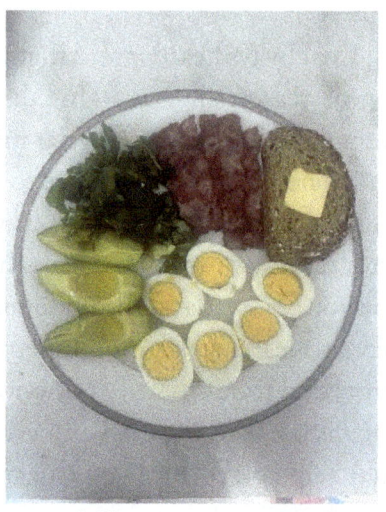

Rye bread toast with avocado and salmon is delicious. You can add peanut butter according to your taste. Scrambled eggs with whole wheat bread. Pudding with chia seeds. Oatmeal with cinnamon plus unsweetened granola with almond milk, among many other options.

Like all diabetics, you should eat every three hours and an ideal snack is a small fruit such as a tangerine, plum, melon, strawberries, apples, bananas, grapes, blueberries, and blackberries, as long as you regulate the portions of these because consuming them in excess can also raise your blood glucose levels. Not only are they delicious, but they are also a great source of vitamin C, necessary for the body, accompanied by some dried fruit. Some fruits with a high glycemic index are pineapple, mango, and raisins, although you can consume them by properly regulating the portions.

Lunch

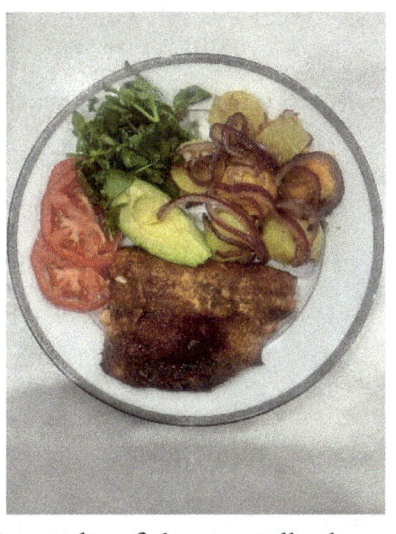

Vegetables are of great importance in your diet. The vegetables that you can add to your balanced diet are lettuce, broccoli, zucchini, chayote, mushrooms, onion, tomato, spinach, cauliflower, eggplant, carrot, paprika, cabbage, and asparagus, among others.

As proteins, you should add skinless chicken or turkey, cuts of fat-free beef, roasts or chops if red meat is still part of your diet, fish, especially those rich in omega-3 fatty acids such as albacore tuna, salmon and also whole eggs consumed during the week, without establishing a maximum per day, but there should be no more than three depending on your weight or preference. In the past, there was a theory that it was not healthy to consume more than seven eggs a week because it supposedly raised your cholesterol. However, nowadays they recommend that we eat it daily because they argue that it is one of the most complete proteins that exists. Its use will depend on the individual preferences of each person.

At Your Dinner

1. **Controlling Your Carb Intake.**
   - Carbohydrates are broken down into glucose, which increases blood sugar levels.

2. **Increase your fiber intake.**
   - Soluble fiber is the most effective for controlling your blood sugar.

3. **Drink plenty of water and stay hydrated.**
   - Remember that 70% of our body is water; consuming enough gives us an adequate balance.

4. **Control daily meal portions.**
   - Measure and weigh your portions. This will only be while you get used to the right portions.
   - Use small plates.
   - Eat slowly.
   - The more control you have over portion sizes, the better control you have over your blood sugar levels.

5. **Choose the right foods with a low glycemic index.**

6. **Manage your stress levels.**

7. **Monitor your blood sugar levels.**
   - Checking your blood sugar with the right technology available today will help you reduce blood sugar spikes and lows; remember that what you measure is controlled.

8. **Eat foods rich in chromium and magnesium.**

    • These are important micronutrients that help control your blood sugar levels.

9. **Add apple cider vinegar to your diet by using it as a dressing in your salads.**

    • The properties of apple cider vinegar help keep your blood sugar levels low.

10. **Get a good enough sleep.**

    • Quality sleep (minimum 8 hours) keeps you under control, while if you sleep poorly, you can interrupt important metabolic hormones that raise your blood sugar levels, especially cortisol, which is elevated due to your poor sleep quality, causing your levels to be not only high but also uncontrolled throughout the day and the next day.

Foods that you definitely need to eliminate from your diet are sugary foods like candy, cookies, cakes, ice cream, sweetened cereals, and canned fruits with added sugar. Also, eliminate drinks with added sugars, such as juices, regular sodas, and regular sports or energy drinks.

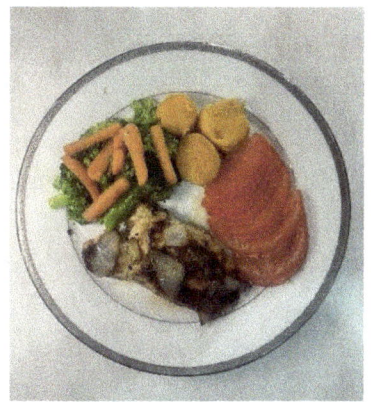

Chapter 5

Your Physical Activity

Maintain an Appropriate Weight. Maintaining a healthy weight will help you manage your diabetes. Exercise regularly.

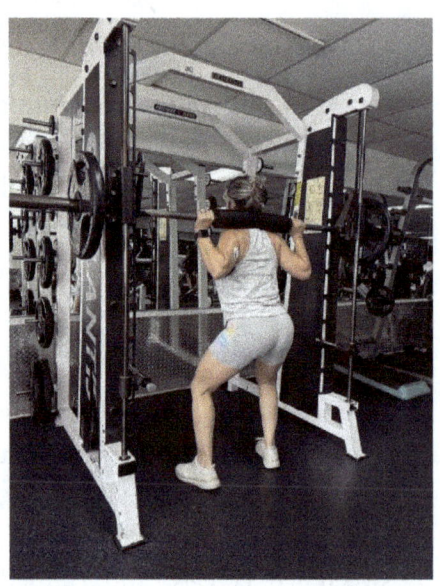

Exercise increases insulin sensitivity and helps your muscles get sugar from your blood. Drink plenty of water and stay hydrated, especially when you're doing physical activity. Remember that 70% of our body is water; consuming enough gives us an adequate balance. Exercise and relaxation methods, such as yoga, will help you stay relaxed.

Monitor your blood sugar levels while exercising because a drop can cause hypoglycemia, which can be very unpleasant, so try to avoid it. When you exercise, always carry a small fruit, a candy, or a sweetened drink with you so that you can quickly recover once you start to feel that your blood sugar is dropping. Remember that it is very dangerous, in addition to hurting your body, not to mention that you could lose consciousness, convulse, etc. But don't worry too much; there's no need to go to that extreme if you take the necessary steps.

Checking your blood sugar with the right technology available today will help you reduce blood sugar spikes and lows; remember that what you measure is controlled. Fortunately, we have a lot of technology available that makes our lives easier.

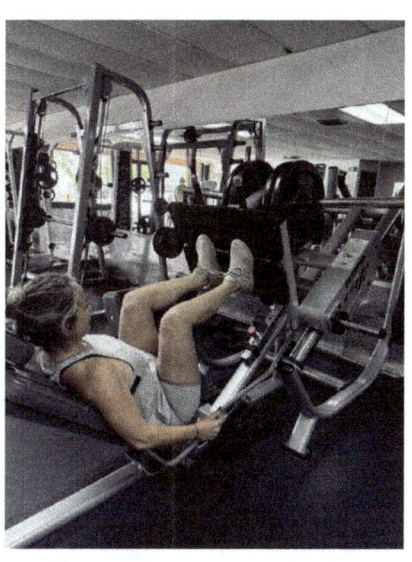

Much more important than doing cardio exercises, you need to work on strength exercises to gain muscle mass. Focus on compound exercises such as squats, deadlifts, and bench presses, which work multiple muscle groups at once. You can also include bodyweight exercises like push-ups and pull-ups, and for the best results, it's crucial to maintain a consistent and progressive training routine, increasing reps or weight over time.

Compound Exercises (With Free Weights or Machines)

- Squats: They work the quadriceps, glutes, and hamstrings.
- Deadlift: Exercises your back, quadriceps, and hamstrings.
- Bench press: Focuses on the chest and triceps.
- Pull-ups: They work the lats, deltoids, and trapezius.
- Dumbbell row: Strengthens the lats and muscles of the arm.

Bodyweight Exercises

- Push-ups (push-ups): They work the shoulders, triceps, and chest.
- Parallel dips: Exercises chest, shoulders, and triceps.
- Jump squats: A more dynamic exercise for quadriceps and glutes.
- Planks: Improve abdominal strength and stability.
- Burpees: A full-body exercise that combines strength and cardio.

Tips To Optimize Muscle Growth

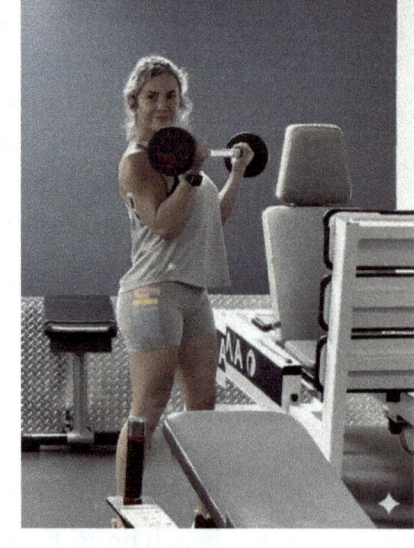

- Progressive overload: Gradually increase the reps, sets, or weight you lift to continue stimulating muscle growth.
- Training frequency: Train each major muscle group about twice a week to encourage further development.
- Cardio exercises are very beneficial, but I particularly do not recommend them because they lower blood sugar levels very quickly. All these strength exercises already include cardiovascular activity, so we don't need more, just the right measure.

Maintain an appropriate weight. Maintaining a healthy weight will help you manage your diabetes. I consider myself a living example that, if you can, striving yourself, fighting day by day with the disease, you can have a full and healthy life like anyone else. Yes, you are going to have some limitations, but this, in turn, will help you have self-control, and you will show the world that you are capable of anything you set your mind to because no one but you has the power to do it.

Below I want to show you some recent graphs that show how my day to day evolves, first in a period of seven days and the second in a period of one month so that you understand that you can live a full life despite the difficulties as long as you do what is indicated. Remember:

1. Take care of your emotional well-being.
2. Maintain a balanced diet.
3. Do regular physical exercise.

This is why I say that I am fortunate to live with diabetes because I have the possibility to be in control of my life in a way. We must never forget the importance of following the instructions of a health professional and using the medications indicated by him. Also, you must remember that everyone is different so it is very important that you listen to your body because what works for others may not work for you in the same way.

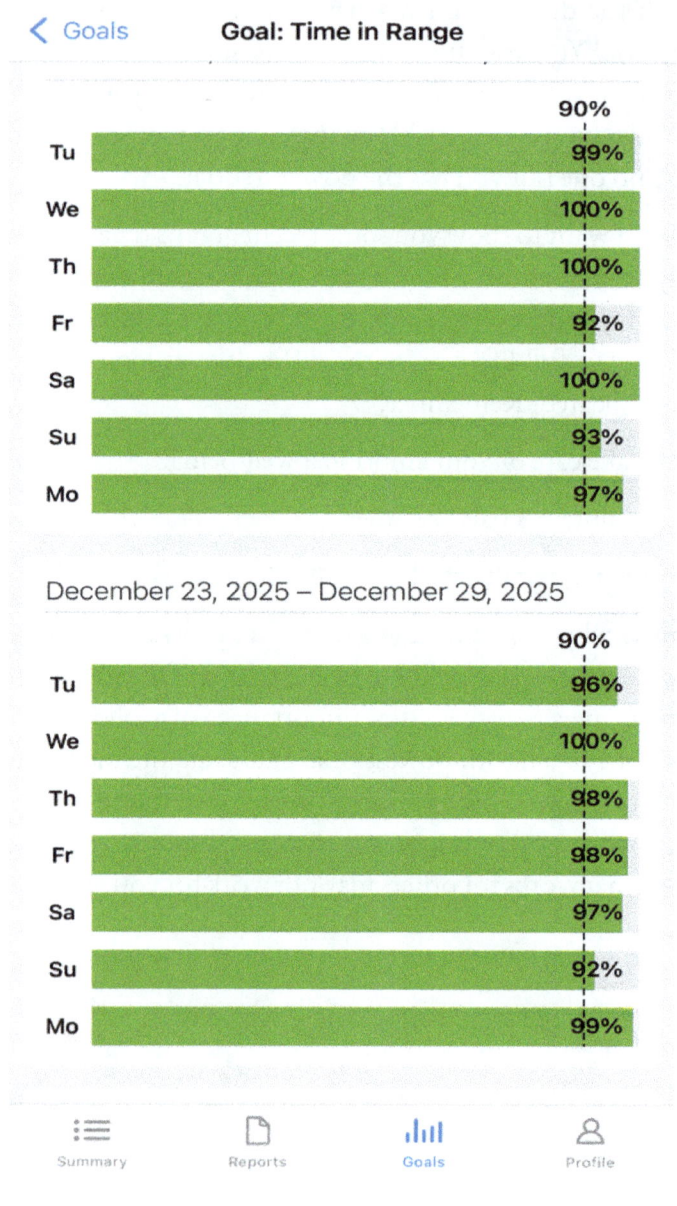

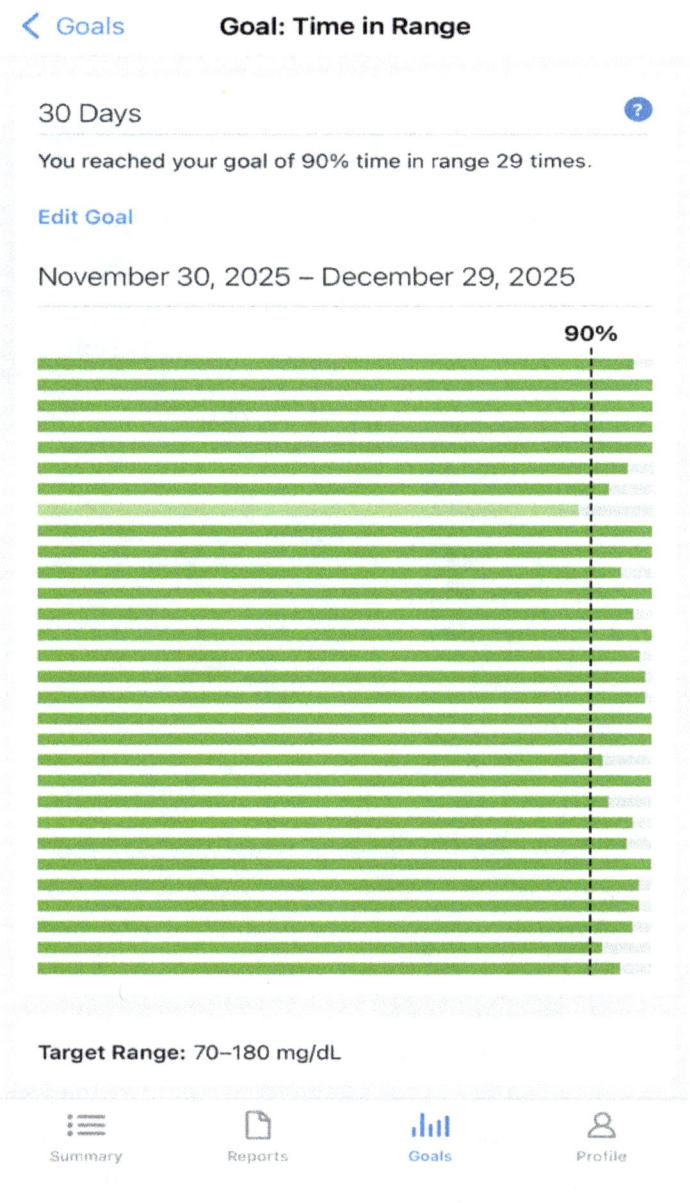

Reflection

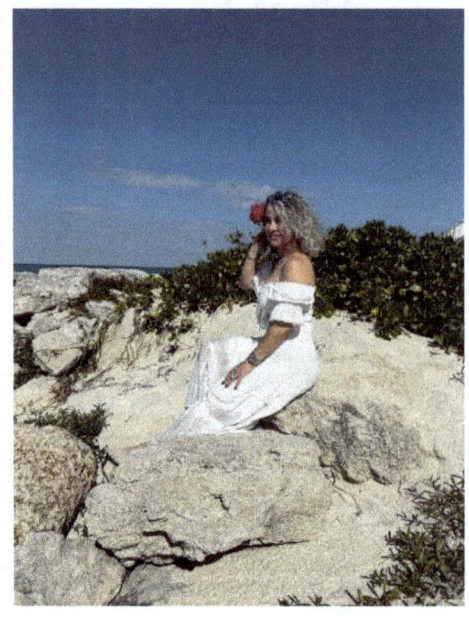

I would not like to end without first reflecting on the important role played by all the people who in one way or another are around us. Diabetes is a manageable disease, if you can live with it, in fact it never leaves you when you sleep, or when you are exhausted, or at parties or if you are sick. Even when you think you're doing everything right, it's not always the case. People don't see your mental exhaustion, your constant insertion for always having to be alert calculating and recalculating. Just because it's a manageable disease doesn't mean it's easy to live with. Surround yourself with people with great empathy either at work, your home, or those companions that we choose to walk our life called friends who cannot be many but you will know that those who choose to stay will be the right ones to walk by your side on this beautiful, turbulent and beautiful path that we call life. If you are fortunate enough to have those valuable people in your life, take care of them as they do with you. We need empathy not to be underestimated, but to understand the courage it takes to stay on your feet despite difficulties.

The day will undoubtedly come. Remembering this as a thing of the past will be very comforting, but as long as this happens, this disease should be treated for what it is, not as a business. The high prices of all the medications necessary to have quality of life living with diabetes are inaccessible to many and this definitely has to change. It is not a luxury, it is a necessity. Guaranteeing this well-being is something that should concern us all because like me and many others it caught us by surprise so it could happen to anyone.

Today I want to thank God for what I am, for what I am not, for what I have and for what I don't have. For having been born where I was born, for having the family I have, for feeling, for remembering, for not forgetting, for what I laugh, for what I cry. FOR BEING ALIVE.

Love life! Revolutionize in the face of difficulties. He resurfaces once again and remembers that the one whom God blesses does not lose, even if he is cheated

www.ingramcontent.com/pod-product-compliance
Lightning Source LLC
Chambersburg PA
CBHW060950050426
42337CB00052B/3508